Gardening Your Way
to
Fitness

I0419568

The Fun Way to Get Fit and Provide Beauty and Healthful Bounty for Your Family

RON KNESS

Contents

Disclaimer

No part of this book may be reproduced, stored in a retrieval system, or transmitted in any form or by any means, electronic, mechanical, photocopying, recording, scanning, or otherwise, without the prior written permission of the publisher.

All the material contained in this book is provided for educational and informational purposes only. No responsibility can be taken for any results or outcomes resulting from the use of this material.

While every attempt has been made to provide information that is both accurate and effective, the author does not assume any responsibility for the accuracy or use/misuse of this information.

The health-related information in this book is meant for informational purposes only. It is not intended to serve as medical advice, substitute for a doctor's appointment or to be used for diagnosing or treating a disease. Readers are advised to consult with their physician before making any decisions concerning their health.

Use this information at your own risk.

Introduction

Gardening is the ultimate exercise model for a healthy and robust lifestyle. When you garden you're getting it all – exercise to positively affect every part of your body; health from being outdoors and breathing in the fresh air; and a lifestyle of creativity, beauty and the joy of being able to reap a harvest of fresh food for your table.

Not all gardeners are fit – some spend the winter months mostly lounging on the sofa while the weather outside is too bad to garden. When the weather changes and it's time to get outdoors again, spring and summer gardeners may suffer from sore muscles and stiff joints 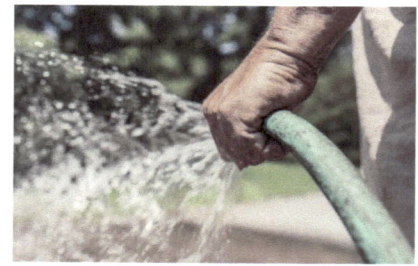 if they don't properly prepare themselves. During the times that being outdoors isn't possible, there are many things you can do to keep your body fit and ready for those garden tasks.

In this guide you'll learn the proper way to stretch and bend and some easy exercises you can do indoors during bad weather days. It's extremely important that you prepare your body (and mind) for the rigorous months of summer gardening.

You'll also learn the three main gardening benefits to your health and fitness – endurance, flexibility and strength. Preparing your body for gardening is similar to preparing to run a marathon. You don't begin to get in shape a week before the marathon – you plan at least a year ahead.

There are some easy, but effective exercises that you can do to prepare your body. Contained in this guide are exercises to benefit the glutes, stretching to make you more flexible and some that are designed to increase your strength. You don't have to have a gym membership or become a body-builder, but keeping your body healthy and fit will be a huge advantage when you begin the gardening process.

Whether you garden for beauty or for food, it's one of the best and most doctor-recommended exercises. Besides being healthy for your body, gardening gives you a new perspective on everything. Seniors that garden have a much lower chance of developing dementia or other chronic diseases as they age.

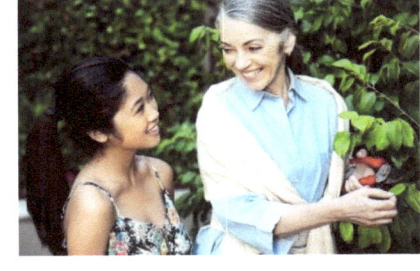

You'll learn about some important studies proving people who garden have lower incidence of everything from depression to heart disease and much more. One very important study showed that seniors who gardened lived much happier and longer lives than their counterparts who didn't garden.

The benefits of gardening are endless. It's good for the body, mind and spirit and can keep you in good health for years. Gardening isn't mindless exercise on a treadmill – it's thinking, plotting and planning your garden so you get the best harvest. It's also hard work. But, when you see the beauty you've created or put food on the table, it's definitely worth the effort.

Improve Your Health Through Gardening

What could be better than feeling the warm sunshine, communing with nature and getting a great overall workout? Gardening provides all that – and more. Your good health will soar when you decide to reap the benefits of gardening – either for the beauty it brings – or the bounty it puts on the table.

When you do it right, you'll get all the exercise you need from gardening. When you're not actually working outdoors, you can perform gardening exercises indoors. Bending, stretching and squatting are all workouts you can get from an expensive gym membership, but why not garden and get even more for your efforts?

Regardless of your age or health, you can get the best workout for your level of fitness by gardening. Even if you only have a patio space, there are plenty of things you can do to improve your health and make your life a bit more enjoyable.

If you have a large garden space, you may want to try growing

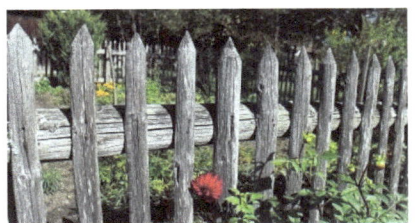 some vegetables – but if you have no interest in that, the beauty which comes from the colorful flowers you can plant will be pleasing to the eye and you can even bring them in for instant decoration. Plus, a garden becomes an instant space for meditation. You can add some elements like a water feature, pond, table and chairs and shade to entice and delight.

Besides the obvious fitness benefits you'll enjoy from gardening, you'll also keep your mind active and sharp. Gardening isn't simply the act of throwing out seeds or planting seedlings in the soil. You've also got to figure out the best place for your plants, how many plants will grow in a certain area, know your soil content and much more.

And, don't forget the lift to your spirit that you'll surely gain from being outdoors, becoming fit and enjoying a hobby which will add more than just plenty of exercise to your life. Get your family involved and multiply the benefits of tending a garden tenfold.

Getting the Most from Your Garden Space

Whether you have acres for planting or a simple patio space, you can get the most exercise and harvest from your garden space if you first research your options. If you're planting in containers, there's lifting, bending, squatting and reaching involved. It's not on the same exercise level as planting a larger space, but it can be super beneficial to your long-term health.

The work begins long before it is time to place the fragile plants or seeds in the soil. Eliminating weeds with hoe or hands and preparing the soil for the plants you've chosen are just a couple of the pre-planting chores on

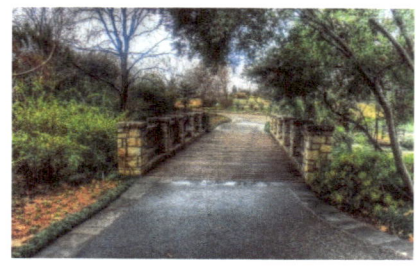

your list. When you spend time and effort preparing your gardening space you'll benefit from both the exercise and the beauty and bounty you reap.

If soil drainage isn't good, you'll need to shore up the soil or build it up to ensure proper drainage. Even if you are gardening in containers, making sure they're clean and hauling soil is exercise you wouldn't be getting while watching television on the sofa.

Before you dive into all the outdoor chores involved in preparing for a garden, you can prepare your body for the gardening chores. Done correctly, a little bit of preventive stretches and other exercises can prevent a ton of aches and pains.

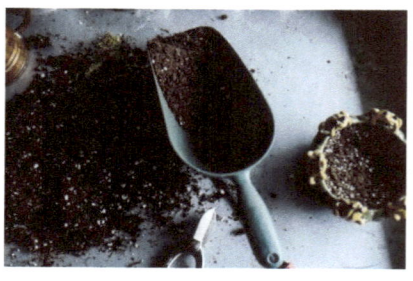

Gardening isn't just about pulling and stretching – this guide will give you some tips to get a good cardio workout while pushing that mower or tiller. Proper tools are a necessity when gardening. You'll also learn which gardening tools will provide the best workout for endurance, flexibility and strength.

The great outdoors is filled with hazards that can't be avoided when working in your garden. Pests such as bugs, poison plants and animals ruining all the work you've put in to your garden. The sun can also be a hazard unless you're well protected.

Lastly, you'll learn what the benefits of gardening are – beyond the healthy environment and exercise. There are benefits to the mind and spirit which can't be explained, but which you'll feel when you enter the amazing and rewarding world of gardening.

Warm Up Your Body Before Starting Gardening Chores

Most people don't begin a marathon race without some stretching and flexing. They may prepare for months before the marathon event to help prevent soreness and injuries -- and to build strength and endurance to ensure victory. You should treat gardening chores the same as you would running a marathon by preparing your body for the tasks ahead.

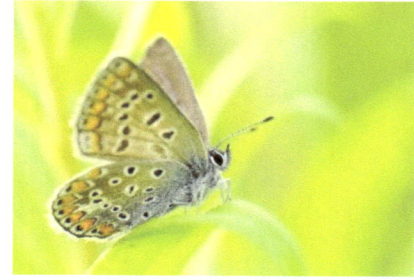

Here are some various exercises which will keep you fit and enhance your gardening experience:

Flexibility

1. **Legs, chest, back and shoulders** – Feet together, knees slightly bent, bend forward and link your fingers behind your back. Distribute your weight evenly; relax the weight on your neck, head and shoulders. Now, lift your arms over your head and bring them perpendicular to the shoulders. Slowly breathe in and out.

2. **Back and shoulders** – Feet together, knees slightly bent, place left hand on left hip and stretch right arm overhead to line up with your ear. Lean left; reach up and left with your right arm while holding stomach in. Repeat for right arm.
3. **Back and chest** – On all fours, place hands apart (shoulder distance) and knees at hip distance. Tighten stomach by pulling navel toward spine. Round back from head to tailbone. Relax and lower your neck and head while exhaling.

Core and Lower Back

1. **Lower back** – Standing with your feet together and hands on hips, lift left leg to the side (exhale) until about 6-inches from floor. Return to beginning position, keeping hips aligned. Repeat with right leg.
2. **Abdomen** – Called a "plie" – begin by standing straight with feet wider than hips. Turn feet slightly out while hands on thighs. Bend knees and lower buttocks while keeping back straight and abdominal muscles tight.
3. **Back and abdomen** – Standing with feet together and hands to side, bend elbows and lift right knee up as much as you can, then go back to beginning stance. Repeat with left knee.

Arms and Shoulders

1. **Arms** – Lying on stomach, lift body to plank position. Place right hand on a ball (such as soccer ball) and left hand on floor and lower your body toward floor, keeping elbows in. Push up again and repeat on the right side.
2. **Shoulders** – Standing position, holding arms straight out and palms up, circle arms forward about 10 times and then backwards 10 times. Turn palms down and repeat the exercise.
3. **Arms/Shoulders** – Jumping jacks will improve both your arms and shoulder strength. Be sure to raise your arms completely above your head when jumping upward.

Glutes

1. **Lower Back and Butt** – Lie on back, arms at sides and feet on floor; Lift hips upward as far as comfortable, tightening your abs and glutes as you lift. Hold for a count and lower back to the floor.
2. **Glutes** – Lie on floor with arms at sides; lift feet so legs are perpendicular to the floor; tap your left foot on the floor slowly and alternate with your left foot for about a minute.
3. **Lower Back/Glutes** – Standing with legs shoulder-length apart, sit back in a squat, bringing fists to chin; extend arms forward and bring leg behind you (straight); return to squatting position and repeat on other side.

The Pre-Gardening Warmup

It's vitally important that you perform some stretching and flexibility exercise just before you exert yourself in the garden. You'll help prevent muscle soreness and joint aches and serious injuries.

Use some of the above exercises for a quick and easy warm up or other flexibility and stretching exercises you're familiar with. You can get into the heavy parts of gardening before you know it – and it's a good thing if your muscles and joints are ready.

Gardening for Seniors

Gardening is the favorite leisure activity for seniors and can keep you healthy and vital well into old age. If you have challenges such as not being able to work on your knees, be sure and use a stool or chair and drink plenty of water outdoors.

Wear lightweight clothing while performing gardening chores – and a hat and sunscreen. It's best to garden early in the morning and avoid the sun and heat of the late afternoon.

Gardening can enrich seniors' lives physically, mentally and spiritually. Joining a gardening club or association may also help the socializing factor of growing older. It's also an activity as light or strenuous as you choose.

Gardening for the Disabled

Gardening isn't just for the robust people in the world – many disabled people love gardening or being in a garden and enjoying the beauty. Some tips to help the disabled enjoy gardening include making paths accommodating a wheelchair and raising the beds to be more accessible. With a little foresight, gardens and gardening can boost the health and spirits of the disabled.

Gain Endurance, Flexibility and Strength From Gardening

Whether you garden for exercise, fun, creating beauty or bounty, you'll be getting the most you possibly can from an exercise routine. You'll get the workout you need to keep your body fit in flexibility, strength and endurance. Research shows that gardening benefits each person, school, home and community in many ways.

There are several exercise benefits of gardening if performed properly. There are three main health benefits you'll enjoy from gardening: endurance, flexibility and strength. You'll be improving your mind and exercising your body for an all-over fitness regime.

Gardening for Endurance

As research on gardening for exercise indicated how beneficial gardening can be for your health, a new term emerged for getting a cardio workout from gardening – aerobic gardening. Aerobic gardening can boost your heart health with workouts including everything from mowing the yard to hauling materials in a wheelbarrow.

Aerobic gardening is a method for gardeners to receive a vigorous workout rather than the stopping or starting in bursts. The continuous movements of aerobic gardening keep the heart rate elevated and the calories burning. In fact, when you spend an hour performing aerobic gardening, it's equal to jogging for four miles.

It's important that you vary the aerobic type of exercises and not spend too much time on one continuous type of exercise. For example, you can spend 10 minutes mowing the yard and then switch to pushing the wheelbarrow or hoeing the weeds from the garden.

If your garden isn't large enough to get enough aerobic exercise, you should practice indoors before you garden. Jumping jacks, running in place or walking on the treadmill can get your cardio rating up. Then, move your exercises to the outdoors where you can build strength and flexibility.

Stretching and Bending for Flexibility

The stretching and bending motions of gardening can give you the flexibility you desire for your body. When you're flexible, you can move your knees and hips easily and your joints will be healthy. Sometimes, you may have great flexibility in one area and less in another.

Flexibility will help you more enjoy the activities you may have given up on in the past. Simple chores such as tying your shoes and having to reach for something will become easier and prevent pain or other discomfort.

It's especially important in your later years that you move with the least amount of discomfort. Keeping your limbs flexible can also help if you need joint surgery at some point in your life and also prevent serious injuries.

Any gentle movement (such as Yoga and Tai Chi) can stretch your muscles and keep you flexible. When you practice stretching before it's time for gardening chores, you'll ensure that you have the flexibility needed for balance, muscle strength and relaxation. When gardening, try slow and gentle movements rather than fast, jerky ones.

Use both sides of the body when gardening and don't stretch to the point of discomfort. As you stretch, watch your breath, making sure you breathe normally – and always include some stretching exercises in your pre-gardening warm-up.

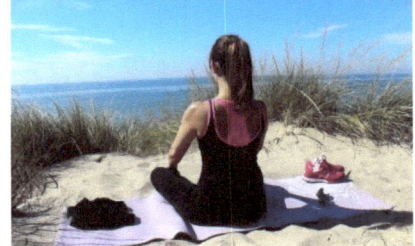

Pushing and Lifting for Strength

Whatever you do in the gardening realm, you'll need a certain amount of strength for the tasks. Pushing a wheelbarrow, lifting boxes and bags are part of the gardening chores which will help you build muscle and joint strength.

Turning a bare piece of land or lawn into planting beds for a vegetable garden requires such tasks as shoveling, raking, pushing wheelbarrows full of materials, bending or squatting to pick up rocks, hoeing weeds and carrying bags. Unless you've built up your strength beforehand, you may find yourself barely able to get out of bed after a day of gardening.

Keep in good physical condition before and during the gardening months by working out to increase your strength as well as your

flexibility and endurance. There are many ways to keep fit – both at home and in the gym. Use weights or kettlebells to strengthen your muscles. Be sure to keep your back and shoulders strong for gardening chores such as hauling heavy loads.

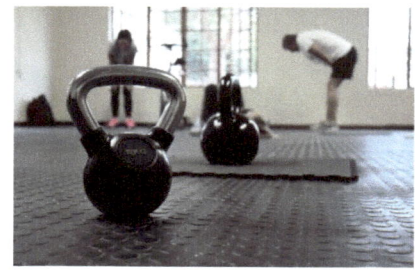

Keeping your body strong before you begin to garden ensures that you'll start with the endurance, flexibility and strength you need for the entire gardening season. You'll be especially glad you did when you can ease into your gardening journey without the inevitability of sore muscles and joints.

The Sun, Overexertion and Pests – Be Aware of the 3 Common Hazards of Gardening

Enjoying the great outdoors and all the benefits it offers is one of the reasons many people begin to garden. But, as with most everything – with the good comes the bad. There are certain hazards of being outdoors and performing the strenuous chores of gardening that could make your joy of gardening turn into a nightmare unless you take necessary precautions.

Here are some tips to prevent gardening hazards:

- **Choose the proper tools for the job**. You should always purchase the best tools you can afford. Even though a certain brand of tool may cost more than a cheap counterpart, the quality will come through in performing the job it's designed for and to prevent possible injury from breakage or slips.
For example, shovels (spades) come designed for many jobs. There is the general garden spade; transplanting spade with a long, narrow blade; border spade for tight spaces and specialty spades for a number of other garden issues.

- **Use sunscreen and wear a hat for sun protection.** Gardening in the warm sun can be such a pleasure – but, if you're not careful you can get into a nightmare of pain and suffering. Broad spectrum SPF 30 sunscreen is a must when you're in the sun for extended periods of time.

After time in the sun, an "after sun" lotion is recommended to protect your skin even more.

A wide-brimmed hat is necessary to protect the sensitive skin of your face. If you burn easily or if it's necessary to be out in the afternoon heat, you should also wear clothing protection such as long-sleeved, lightweight shirts.

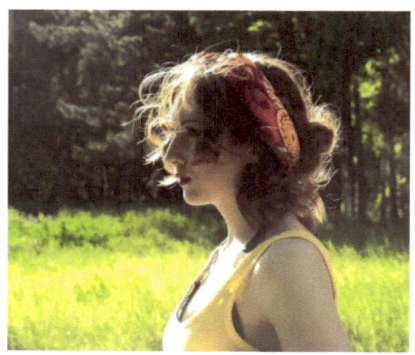

- **Snakes, bugs and poison plants.** Depending on your geographical location, you may need to protect yourself from any or all of these gardening hazards. During hot months, snakes may frequent your garden space looking for water.

Various bugs such as wasps and mosquitos can also make your life miserable in the outdoors unless you take precautions such as wearing boots and remembering to spray yourself with bug repellent. You should know how to identify poison ivy and other poisonous plants and avoid them when you garden.

You don't have to use fertilizers and other harsh chemicals. There are many organic and earth-friendly products which can lower the bug, poison plant and snake population.

- **Hydrate with plenty of water.** Prevent sunstroke and fatigue by keeping yourself hydrated with plenty of water.

Other beverages such as soda and alcohol don't do the job of hydrating your body that water does. Carry a water bottle designed to fit on your belt so you'll have it at all times while you're performing gardening chores.

Many avid gardeners have learned the hard way that too much sun can take a painful toll. At the least, you could suffer from sunburn and the risk of skin cancer – at the worst; you might find yourself in the midst of sunstroke.

- **Take breaks.** It's important that you take time to smell the roses you may have planted – or, at least have a seat and rest while surveying your garden domain. One trait that most gardeners have is that they tend to get carried away when they're enjoying themselves and work way beyond their physical limits. You may want to set a timer to alert you when you've been working for a certain amount of time. Relax with a cool glass of water and begin again when rested.

Your garden is the perfect place to completely relax with a book or glass of wine if you plan it properly. Water features and flower-laden pots, along with a comfortable outdoor chair can be just the place you need to meditate and enjoy life.

- **Vary the chores.** Don't spend your entire time in the garden performing one type of task. Spending too much time on one chore requiring a certain set of muscles can wreak havoc afterward. Sore muscles and joint pain are often the results of gardeners getting carried away and wanting to get the job done regardless of the time involved. Take it easy and don't overdo one set of muscles – vary your gardening chores.

Also, be sure that you expend energy on both sides of the body. If you're right-handed, you may have a sore shoulder or arm from pulling weeds while exclusively using that arm. Use your less predominant arm and hands just as much as the dominant one.

- **Safety first.** All outdoor activities require that you practice safety first by taking the proper precautions. Protecting your skin against the sun's harmful rays is one way to be safe in the garden. You may want to consider hiring a contractor to handle jobs requiring skills such as using a chainsaw. Minimally, watch some training videos or pay a skilled professional for a few hours of training.
Your local home improvement store may have videos you can borrow to learn how to do a number of garden chores (and indoor chores) safely and which equipment will be the best for the job.

If you can avoid it, don't work alone – or at least without telling someone where you'll be when you're working outdoors. Ideally, there should be two or more people when working in the garden and especially when climbing ladders and operating special equipment.

When you have to work in the garden alone, be sure that you have a mobile phone or other type of device so that you can immediately contact someone if an emergency occurs.

Harvesting More Than Produce – The Benefits of Gardening That Go Beyond Raising Vegetables and Flowers

You've got to spend some months preparing for its arrival, making sure the soil it grows in is nutritious and healthy – plus, devote your undivided attention to keeping it healthy and growing after it's planted. But, the rewards are enormous. Not only will you gain robust health and vitality from gardening, but you'll also reap the beauty and/or bounty of what you've nurtured.

Gardening for Clarity and Knowledge

A quote from John Burroughs, an American naturalist and writer, says it all: "I go to nature to be soothed and healed, and to have my senses put in tune once more." Being in the outdoors and communing with nature has benefits far beyond the obvious. It also promotes mental health by providing relaxation and the satisfaction of having created something you can be proud of.

Research indicates that seniors (those people over 60 years of age) who garden on a regular basis have an almost 40% less chance of developing dementia than those who don't garden. This research also takes into consideration other health factors which may contribute to dementia.

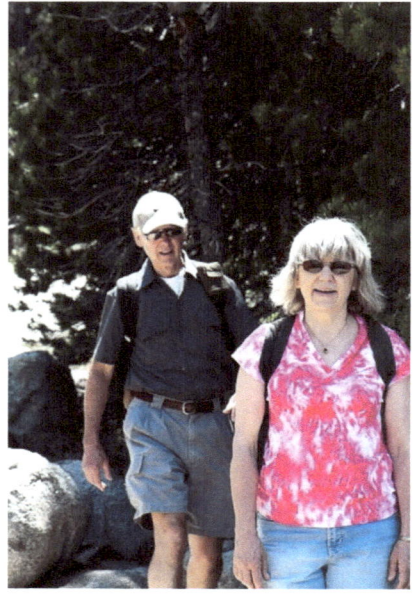

Another factor in gardening for mental health is that a harmless bacterium called Mycobacterium found in soil can stimulate the immune system and boost your serotonin levels. Serotonin is a chemical produced by the brain which regulates your moods. If your serotonin levels are low, you have a greater risk of developing depression. Working with the soil can help to elevate your moods and keep you from becoming depressed.

Research has also found that those who garden enjoy a more positive outlook on life and are happier than those who don't garden. Vitality and mental acuity are also improved in people who garden on a regular basis.

Gardening isn't all work – you must also think and be creative. This keeps your mind active and can protect you against many diseases. When you keep your mind active and thinking, you'll likely avoid many maladies preventing you from enjoying your later years.

Gardening for the Spirit

Gardening can also be good for the spirit by providing a soothing place of your own to relax, reflect and restore your peace of mind – a place where the beauty and colors of nature are perfect to watch and learn new things.

The cycles of nature coincide with the rhythms of our lives and when we garden, our minds become engrossed with what we're doing worries seem to evaporate. That's exactly why gardening is a good way to escape from the stresses of the world. When you reduce stress, you're also reducing the likelihood of developing stress-caused medical problems such as anxiety, heart disease and high blood pressure.

Sound and touch are also a part of garden's healing properties.

Hearing the rustling of leaves in the wind can be soothing as can running water in a garden's pond or water feature. The tactile sense can also benefit. When you touch velvety leaves or rose petals, you're enjoying the moment of softness and fragility.

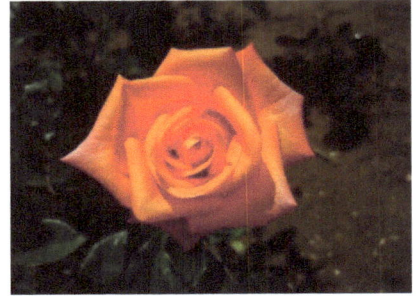

When you look at a nature scene, your spirit is restored, whereas looking at a city scene full of concrete and steel is found to cause anxiety. Herbs can be especially helpful to renewing the senses. Rosemary, basil and thyme are herbs which are gifts that keep on giving – both in the kitchen and for our health.

Gardening for Beauty and Food

The garden is a sensory place where all five senses are stimulated. It provides a kaleidoscope of colors are calming and also gives us produce with wonderful tastes and textures.

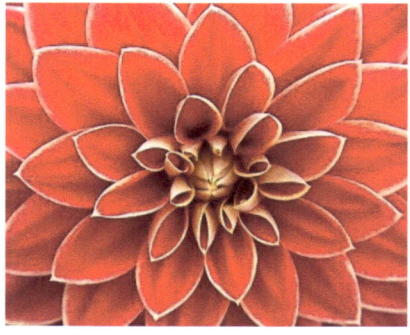

Aromatic herbs such as mints can be both pleasing to the eye and produce a wonderful scent. You can also use them in the kitchen. Flowers go beyond the beauty they provide and can be elements to use for décor in your home. They can also provide a pleasing place in which to relax and meditate.

If you choose to plant a vegetable garden, you'll enjoy a pleasing new freshness to your taste over those you purchase in a supermarket. Satisfaction is also a factor when you grow your own food. You'll be saving money as well as enjoying an adventure that your entire family can participate in.

Which vegetables you grow depends on the area in which you live, but some of the most popular and resilient vegetables include tomatoes, okra, lettuce, eggplant and squash. Try growing some fruit in your garden too, such as watermelon, cantaloupe and other fruits indigenous to your area.

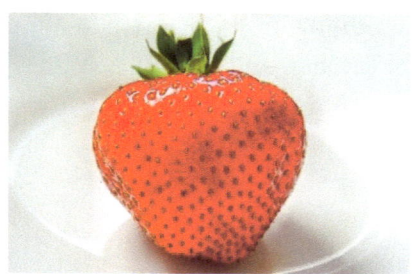

Gardening for Satisfaction and Quality of Life

Rounding up all the benefits of gardening, satisfaction and increasing the quality of life are also advantages. Those who are 50 years of age and older often garden for the satisfaction they get from tending a vegetable or flower garden, the exercise and the lifting of the spirit.

There are many compelling reasons to add gardening to your life's activities, but as you grow older, these reasons become even more compelling and the positive impact on senior's lives is profound. Those seniors over 65 years of age who garden are said to be at much less risk of developing chronic diseases.

Today, gardening has become one of the most popular leisure activities to those adults over the age of 65. The attitudes and health of older gardeners are much improved over those who don't garden. The Life Satisfaction Inventory A is a tool measuring the quality of life according to five components:

1. "Resolution and Fortitude"
2. "Zest for Life"
3. "Physical, Psychological, and Social Self-Concept"
4. "Congruence Between Desired and Achieved Goals"
5. "Optimism"

Researchers used the tool to measure the health and attitudes of 298 participants who were divided into those who defined themselves as "gardeners or non-gardeners." They found that there were substantial differences in the participants overall satisfactions with their lives.

The more positive results were associated with those seniors who defined themselves as gardeners and over 84% had made future plans compared to just 68% of non-gardeners. Also, most gardeners felt more energetic and vital than those who didn't garden.

There have been many studies which present strong facts that gardening is an effective method for all adults – especially those over 50 years of age – to increase the satisfaction they find in life and to get much needed physical activity to reduce chronic illnesses and diseases.

Gardening for a Purpose

Whether you garden for exercise, beauty, food or quality of life, if you want to be successful, you must give it the attention it needs. You can't get by with skipping garden chores like you can wake up one morning and decide you won't go to the gym that day.

When it's time for preparing, planting and harvesting, you need to be ready to meet the challenge. Plan and create a garden design which will effectively meet your wants and needs.

You may want to begin small and expand as your physical strength and stamina improve. As your flair for this incredible hobby increases, so will your desire to do more, plant more, be outdoors more.

Gardening joys and benefits are unlimited and even beginners can appreciate the pursuit of making the earth burst with beauty and bounty – and the affect it has on your body and lifelong health.

Legal Notice

The Publisher has strived to be as accurate and complete as possible in the creation of this book, notwithstanding the fact that he does not warrant or represent at any time that the contents within are accurate due to the rapidly changing nature of the Internet.

The Publisher will not be responsible for any losses or damages of any kind incurred by the reader whether directly or indirectly arising from the use of the information found in this publication.

This book is not intended for use as a source of legal, business, accounting or financial advice. All readers are advised to seek services of competent professionals in legal, business, accounting, and finance field.

No guarantees of income are made. Reader assumes responsibility for use of information contained herein. The author reserves the right to make changes without notice. The Publisher assumes no responsibility or liability whatsoever on the behalf of the reader of this book.

This book may contain affiliate programs and advertisements for monetization, which can result in commissions or advertising fees being earned for purchases made by visitors that click through any of the advertisements and/or links included in this text.

About the Author

I grew up in Central Minnesota, where my parents own and operated a fishing resort. Once out of high school I tried a couple of semesters of college, only to quit halfway through the Spring term; I decided at that time that college wasn't for me.

Then I decided to follow my father's previous occupation as an auto mechanic. I graduated from a two-year of vocational training course and worked as a mechanic. While in vocational training, I decided to join the National Guard where I eventually ended up working full-time for 32 years.

So how does all of this relate to writing? In one of my leadership schools, the instructor, who was an English teacher at a juvenile detention center, presented writing to me in a whole new way - a way that started to develop my interest in working with words.

Fast forward about 40 years and I now have over 20 books listed on Amazon for Kindle. All of my books with the exception of one children's book (One, Two, Three, Four . . . Counting is Fun at the Grocery Store) are non-fiction in various fields, such as:

*Health and Fitness:

- What You Eat Can Hurt You

- Eat Healthy to Lose Weight

- The Extreme Weight Loss Plan

- Get Ripped Abs

- Don't Be In the Dark About Light

- The No Nonsense Guide to Digital Photography

- The Beginner's Guide to Digital Photography

- Digital Photography – A Quick Guide to Using Adobe Photoshop Elements

- Improve Your Blog Posts With Photos

- Digital Photography Anthology

* Travel:
- Travel Advisor

- Travel Trips and Tips

*Outdoors and Recreation:

- Making Your First Fly Rod

- The Beginner's Guide to Fly Tying

- Hooked on Fly Fishing

- The Secrets to Fly Fishing for Trout

- Tent Camping – The Ultimate in Family Fun

- Maintaining a Salt Water Pool

* Misc.:
- Making Wine from Kits

- Create Your Home Inventory

- The 9 Secrets to Using Your GI Bill Benefits

- [The Life and Times of the Honey Bee](#)

- [The Military Spouses Financial Guide to Funding Education](#)

- [The Home-Based Entrepreneur's Guide to Blogging](#)

- [Survival Basics – Are You Prepared to Survive?](#)

Besides my own writing, I also ghostwrite ebooks, reports, articles, blogs and do Kindle conversions for my clients.

Oh . . . did I mention that I went back to college in 1987 and graduated 7 years later?

Today my wife and I live in Gold Canyon, AZ, where you'll find me happily sitting in my office typing away on my laptop as I work on my next book or ghostwriting project . . . that is if we are not traveling on a cruise ship - our new-found mode of travel.

If you like my book, please leave a review.

www.ingramcontent.com/pod-product-compliance
Lightning Source LLC
Chambersburg PA
CBHW050907290526
45792CB00002B/726